The Book of

Nei Kung

The Book of
Nei Kung

C. K. Chu

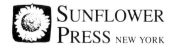

SUNFLOWER
PRESS NEW YORK

First Printing 1986
Second Printing 1996
Third Printing 2007

Library of Congress Cataloging-in-Publication Data

Chu, C.K., 1937-
    The Book of Nei Kung

Chi Kung. I. Title.
GV505.C528   1985   613.7'1   86-23391
ISBN 0-9616586-0-6
ISBN 0-9616586-1-4

10 9 8 7 6 5 4 3

Distributed by
    CHU TAI CHI
    156 West 44th Street • New York, NY 10036
    T: (212) 221-6110   F: (718) 830-9616

Visit our website: www.chutaichi.com

SUNFLOWER PRESS • P.O. Box 750733 • Forest Hills Station • NY 11375-0733

About the Author

Born in 1937, Master C. K. Chu began his study of the martial arts as a youth in Hong Kong. In 1973 he founded his own martial arts studio in Times Square, New York, and has been teaching six days a week ever since at the world-famous Chu Tai Chi school (www.chutaichi.com). In 2000 he also founded the non-profit Tai Chi Chuan Center (www.taichichuancenter.org) to bring the benefits of Tai Chi and Nei Kung to senior centers and parks around New York City.

Sifu Chu holds an M.A. in Physics (City University of New York) and is a retired New York City public school teacher who taught physics at Brooklyn Technical High School, as well as Queens College (C.U.N.Y.) and the New York Institute of Technology. His insights into Nei Kung and Tai Chi are colored by his background in both western science and eastern philosophy.

Master Chu is also the author of "Tai Chi Chuan Principles and Practice" (1981), "Chu Meditation" (2002) and "Eternal Spring Chi Kung" (2003), as well as multiple training DVD's. For more information, including demonstration videos, visit www.chutaichi.com.

Acknowledgments

A path, it is said, is made with the footsteps of many people. The Book of Nei Kung has evolved in much the same way. Of the many students and friends who contributed their valuable time and talents, I especially wish to thank Jim Borrelli and John Shramko. Jim Borrelli was a major driving force from the very beginning. His help in conceptualizing and writing this work has been indispensable. An equally vital role was performed by John Shramko who, in addition to his help in writing, was responsible for the comprehensive organization of the material from the text to the photo strips. Without the unflagging spirit, energy and dedication of John and Jim this book could not have been accomplished.

I also wish to express my appreciation to Kip Meyer for providing the fine photographs, Hing Yin Chu for illustrations, June Jackson for art direction and layout, Tim O'Meara, Richard Marchione and Bob Lyons for typographic assistance and advice, and Robert Anderson, Philip Tartaglia and Marilyn Seiler for critical evaluation. I feel very fortunate to have worked with such generous and gifted people.

Lastly, I am deeply grateful to my family who made my concern for this book their concern too—especially my wife, Carol, for her help with production and proofreading, and my daughter, Elizabeth, for the cover design.

For my daughter, Elizabeth

Contents

Part I—The Essence

Introduction

My philosophy of physical and mental development can be reduced to the basic Taoist principle: "Go with nature and improve what you have." Within these simple words lie the secrets with which one can restructure the mind and body. I believe the two must be in harmony when one reaches for the highest attainable goals.

This book presents a unique set of exercises designed to achieve such ends. Though labeled "exercises", they should not be interpreted in the strict Western sense of the word, for what I am about to discuss constitutes the fundamentals of a system of health which addresses the overall natural ordering of the human body.

This system, known as Nei Kung, has been organized, refined and handed down from master to master through several thousand years of Chinese Taoist tradition. Furthermore, Nei Kung provides the foundation for internal martial arts training. Nei Kung is not the creation of any one teacher. What I have done is to synthesize and group together ten of its simplest forms which are suitable for the average person and from which he or she can gain considerable benefit.

These exercises or postures can be performed by anyone at virtually any age. They have been designed to develop your natural assets. Your body is a highly sophisticated machine. Nei Kung will keep it tuned so that it will operate at optimum levels of efficiency. Nei Kung deals specifically with the flow of energy in the body. You will feel this energy almost at once. In fact, the older you are the faster you will feel the effects of Nei Kung training.

Currently there are numerous conflicting theories about exercise, and people are at a loss as to what is worthwhile to learn and what to discard as fad. One has only twenty-four hours each day. You need to sleep and eat, work and develop your mind. What form of exercise can you fit into your schedule? What will give you the most benefit? The public is understandably confused by differing methods of attaining physical health. Muscle-building machines? Jogging? Aerobics? Most of these forms of exercise do have some beneficial effect on the body but as a whole they do not address the most important problems. The Book of Nei Kung will offer a structured program for the general enhancement of physical fitness, longevity and increased energy for any activity from mental or physical labor to sex and artistic expression.

In my opinion, the disadvantages of traditional Western exercises far outweigh the advantages. From the amateur weekend jogger to the professional athlete injuries abound, all stemming from an incomplete understanding and an improper use of the body.

The individual who is familiar with Nei Kung gradually becomes more aware of his or her body, not only its physical appearance but its inner dynamics as well. When you are in touch with your body, you sense its limitations as well as its potential and, consequently, avoid pushing it beyond its limits. This notion is a fundamental departure from the numerous exercise fads continually thrust upon the public. Weight reduction and tightened muscles do not necessarily constitute sound health.

The practice of Nei Kung will seem odd to many people at first. Yet, very soon, indeed almost at once, something will be felt that is exceptionally pleasant. There will be a flow of warmth through the limbs or perhaps a tingling sensation. For others, a lightness of movement will result, accompanied by a marked release of tension. These are all manifestations of the stimulation of the internal energy or life force of the body. This is "chi." The cultivation and accumulation of chi is the essence of Nei Kung.

The accumulation of chi in the body can be likened to the accumulation of money: the more you have, the more you can spend. You can acquire a very high reserve of chi for use in many activities. Conversely, you can exhaust your chi and be, in effect, physically bankrupt. Chi, like money, has to be earned through work.

This book will present both the theory of Nei Kung and its application. Theory is important in opening the door to understanding this system. This book has been structured to proceed from thought to action. Careful study will allow you to learn by yourself.

You can do so in the privacy of your own home and you will profit every day. Each time you execute these forms, you improve your body and increase your level of chi. The more chi you have, the more you will be able to accomplish in all areas of your life.

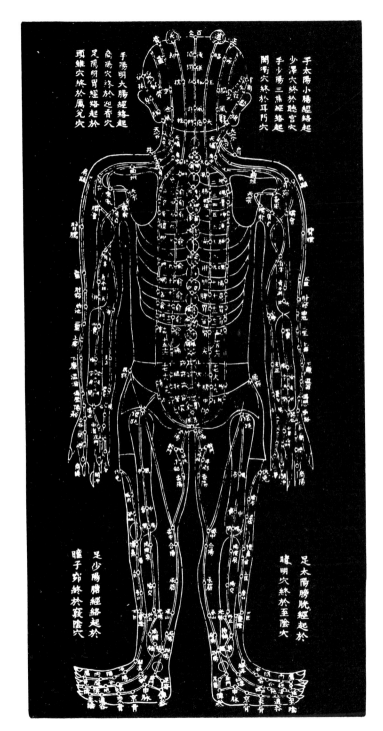

Fig. 1. Meridian Diagram

What Is Nei Kung?

Nei Kung exercises work directly with the chi energy to integrate and strengthen the physical elements of the body: the muscles, the tendons, the bones, the organs, the blood circulation, and the breathing process.

The concept of chi has been utilized for generations by Chinese practitioners of acupuncture and acupressure. It is a physical phenomenon that is believed to be intrinsically present in all life. In one sense, chi is perhaps akin to water in that it can manifest itself as a dynamic flow. The elaborate meridian diagrams (Figure 1) used as the basis for Oriental medical treatments have resulted from considerable practical experience which supports this analogy. Only recently have the tools of modern technology even attempted to probe the specific scientific principles involved. However, the reproducibility of these phenomena over the centuries supports the truth of these claims.

For our purposes, we are more interested in what chi does than in how it does it. A Nei Kung posture both increases the amount of chi available and removes obstacles to its smooth circulation. Again, using the analogy of water, Nei Kung is the "master irrigator" of the body. The channels are dug, the water (energy) is produced and is distributed throughout.

While performing a Nei Kung exercise with slow, relaxed breathing, the specific alignment of the body parts creates the necessary conditions to produce chi. A greater supply of chi results in an increased level of vitality and health within the body system. It is quite a radical approach when contrasted with the more familiar routines like jogging or aerobics, which work primarily on the cardiovascular system, or weight lifting, which builds only localized muscular strength. Since Nei Kung works directly with the flow of the life force, it can induce subtle changes on a cellular level.

While Nei Kung is considered an internal system of physical development, the cultivation of chi can also be approached externally, as with the "Eight Bouquet" exercises or the "Five Animal Games" of the early Taoist physical disciplines. The external approach attempts to "pump" chi into the body, while the internal system stresses the body in a specific manner so as to create a chi "vacuum", as it were, that permits the body to absorb more chi naturally. The external approach uses heavy breathing and rapid diaphragmatic exercises, emphasizing concentration and will power to achieve its goals. The internal system employs slow, deep breathing, making the body work like a squeezed sponge, expanding powerfully, thereby increasing the body's capacity to soak up the energy automatically. A major advantage of the internal approach is that blockages in chi flow are opened up gently without applying force which can be damaging to the body.

History of Nei Kung

Nei Kung dates back to the beginning of Chinese history. It was developed and practiced mostly by early Taoists. It predates the Yellow Emperor period (2696-2598 BC), the beginning of Chinese written history. From this period we have related literature that includes meditation, internal organ massage, acupressure and acupuncture. Our interest here is only in the realm of Nei Kung training, however.

In the beginning, certain exercises were recognized as beneficial for the body. Some were developed by observing the movements of various animals, such as tigers, deer, monkeys, bears and cranes. People recognized that different types of animals developed specialized talents and wanted to learn the best from each: the agility of the monkey, the power of the bear, the longevity of the turtle. All of these exercises are based on observed phenomena, the way of nature, and are not arbitrarily invented techniques.

Throughout history, Chinese scholars have tended to pursue the theory of Taoism and have neglected its physical aspect. A scholar traditionally received greater status than a Kung Fu artist. Due to this bias, Nei Kung was not well publicized, even in China itself. Parents would often encourage their children to pursue intellectual disciplines to the detriment of physical exercise. We now realize that the mind performs most efficiently in an active, healthy body.

As a result, these esoteric physical disciplines remained confined to a relatively small group of teachers. Some information leaked out into the general awareness of society, such as the "Eight Bouquet" exercises or the "Eight Treasures." Others were less well known or were kept secret. The transmission of these secrets depended on the handing down from teacher to student over the centuries. As in any oral tradition, mistakes and reinterpretations can occur. Sometimes teachers kept Nei Kung techniques from beginning students because, if not done properly, Nei Kung could be damaging to the body. Consequently, there are virtually no books on the subject.

In times past, learning Kung Fu was considered a matter of survival, not just health. If you did not know how to fight, you could be in trouble at any time. Villages and towns would engage Kung Fu masters to train their own clans. Especially talented pupils were selected to study the Nei Kung system. An advanced student could spend up to three years perfecting just the Embracing Horse stance.

Basics

These are the fundamental principles of body alignment for the forms, presented in order of importance. Each of these principles will be illustrated and explained on the following pages.

1) Head suspended

2) Pelvis tucked in, toe in and knee out

3) Chest concave

4) Body rounded

5) Shoulders and elbows lowered

6) Waist loose

7) "Qua" loose

8) Deep breathing

These basic principles are the points that must be executed correctly at all times. They are the important details that students must be aware of in order to get the maximum benefit and avoid injury. All of these alignments must be correct at the same time so that the body will be pulled and stretched in the appropriate places to stimulate chi circulation. If any one principle is violated, everything will be affected—balance, integration, chi flow—and the exercise becomes essentially useless. This list will serve as a blueprint for students to check themselves. All of these principles must be understood fully before a long term workout program can be effective.

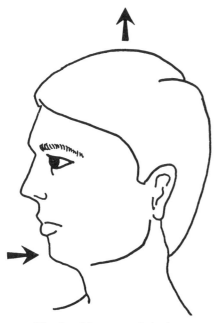

The head is suspended, the eyes gaze forward, and the chin is slightly withdrawn.

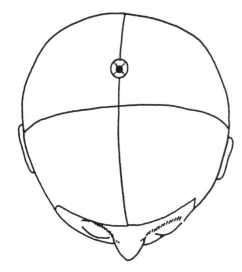

Point of suspension

1) Head suspended

Your body should be suspended as if a string were lifting you by the top of your head. The point of suspension is in the center and towards the rear, as if the spine continued through the skull. When the head is suspended and the shoulders and elbows are lowered, a minimum of energy is being used to maintain an erect posture. Dropping the head or collapsing the shoulders forward will obstruct the flow of chi in the body. A properly suspended head does not tilt backward either. The eyes should be directed ahead with the chin slightly tucked in. The lips should touch, with the teeth gently meshed together. The front upper surface of the tongue should rest on the roof of the mouth, just behind the front teeth. Saliva can then easily flow into the throat.

Suspending the body properly permits the internal organs to sink down or hang in a position of minimal stress. The entire body is in a loose, relaxed, and neutral posture. I must emphasize that loose, in this context, does not mean limp; rather it refers to a quality which incorporates both flexibility and strength—as in the movement of a snake. The Chinese term for this dynamic is "jou" (see C.K. Chu's "T'ai Chi Ch'uan Principles and Practice", p. 169).

2) Pelvis tucked in, toe in and knee out.

"Tucking in the pelvis" is fundamental to all sophisticated martial arts systems. It refers to a forward rotation of the pelvis (as shown in the diagram) which eliminates the hollow in the lower back. Another way of sensing the tucked in position is to imagine you are sitting on an invisible stool while keeping your back straight. Tucking in facilitates a solid root, which means letting the body sink down into a stable stance. It also improves circulation and reduces stress on the lower spine.

"Toe in and knee out" means slightly pushing the knees outward and pulling the toes inward in such a manner as to create a tension in the tendons of the legs thus focusing most of the body weight on the heels and outer edges of the feet (refer to diagram). The inside edges of the feet can be raised off the ground, if necessary, depending on the structure of the individual's foot. This aspect of alignment enhances the stability of the lower body.

I must stress that if you just "tuck in" without "toe in and knee out" you can do yourself more harm than good. When executed in unison, these three elements will begin to produce involuntary breathing from the diaphragm.

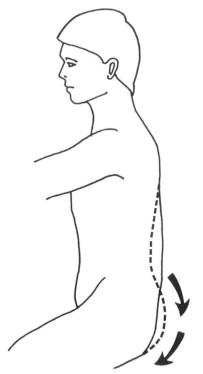

A tucked in pelvis straightens the back.

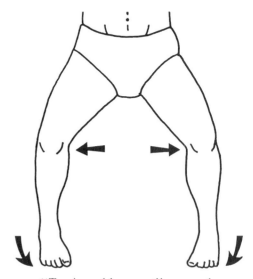

"Toe in and knee out" means the knees are directly over the toes.

3) Chest concave

When you form your chest into a concave shape (refer to diagram), you will induce a downward flow of chi from the front of your chest to the tan tien (the major energy reservoir of the body, located within the abdomen and about two inches below the navel). If you can achieve deep relaxation coupled with tucking in and sinking down, it will induce a flow rising up from the lower back to the top of the head. The downward and upward movement of chi will gradually generate a constant current which we call the Large Orbit. This internal energy circulates from as low as the coccyx to the top of the head and runs down the face and chest, back to the tan tien. It is the "treasure" which many discuss but few achieve.

A concave chest has the form of a semi-circle.

4) Body rounded

Your body should assume a spherical form as opposed to an angular or stiff-limbed configuration. Such is often the case with more conventional calisthenics, which lock the limbs and hyperextend the joints. Roundness of the chest, arms, and hands builds the strongest connections between these elements. Roundness of the lower body is related to "tuck in, toe in, knee out," and helps to improve circulation and physical stability.

Roundness builds the strongest connections.

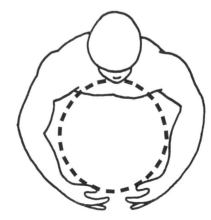

24

5) Shoulders and elbows lowered

You must drop your shoulders and elbows to ensure roundness and relaxation. This also helps your entire body to sink down which, in turn, stabilizes the stance. However, do not slump your shoulders forward.

6) Waist loose

Your waist should be able to twist freely and independently with your legs solidly rooted. Underdeveloped muscles in this area will make this movement difficult, as will overdeveloped muscles which lack flexibility. The "Rhinoceros Gazes at the Moon" posture will help you to develop this important feature (see page 56).

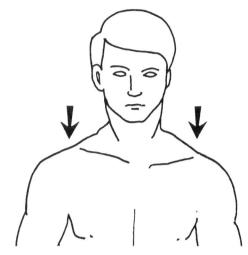

Lowering the shoulders completes the linkage between the arms and the body.

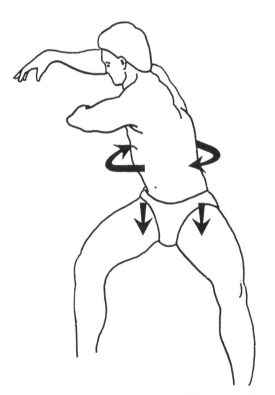
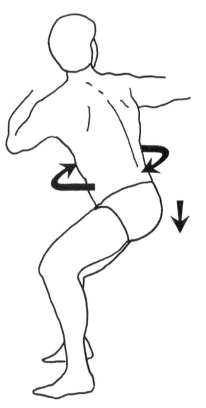

The waist twists freely while the hips, legs, and feet are fixed firmly to the ground.

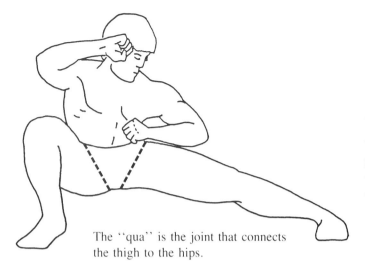

The "qua" is the joint that connects the thigh to the hips.

7) "Qua" loose

The "qua" is the joint that connects the thigh bone and the pelvic bone. (Refer to the dotted line in the diagram.) Stiff tendons will create problems here. With age, this area tends to become even more constricted. Part of the Nei Kung technique will loosen up this vital region to ensure unobstructed circulation of chi. Note, in particular, the "Hitting the Tiger" posture (see page 66).

8) Deep breathing

Proper breathing technique is an essential component of Nei Kung. Each breath should consist of a small flow of air drawn in through the nose by deeply extending the diaphragm in a smooth and uninterrupted manner for a longer duration than normal breathing. The key words to remember are: small, deep, smooth and long. A full extension of the diaphragm expands the lungs completely. The rib cage and chest hardly move during this deep breathing. Instead, the abdomen expands and contracts slightly, as in the diagram.

A few exercises specifically call for a more rapid breathing rate, as in the advanced portion of "Double Dragons Leap from Sea" (see page 52). Deep and smooth breathing through the nose still applies in those cases.

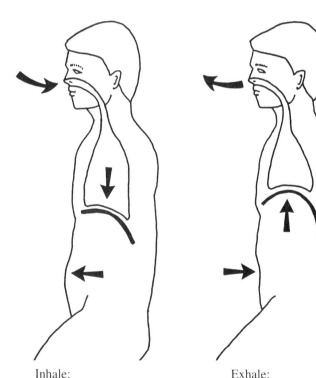

Inhale:
    diaphragm down
    air in
    abdomen out

Exhale:
    diaphragm up
    air out
    abdomen in

Mental Principles

Nei Kung encompasses both physical and mental training. If you underestimate the difficulty involved in either aspect you will only invite failure. Accepting the difficulties involved is the first step. If you succeed in accepting the challenge you will ultimately find, as the Chinese say, the Eternal Youth of the body. In other words, you will slow down the aging clock of your metabolism.

As you prepare for a Nei Kung training session, your mind should be completely at ease. Before the first exercise, you should stand still for a few moments with the head suspended. This orients and relaxes the mind. The pulse and heart beat will soon follow. You are trying to reduce stress so that the entire body will benefit from the flow of energy.

The beginner will experience discomfort in different parts of the body when he or she commences the exercises. You should ask yourself, "Am I doing the posture correctly? Are my knees properly placed?" Adjust yourself as you go along. At no time should you hold your breath. The beginner, especially, should understand that no one can do the postures accurately right away. Some postures may take as long as five years to receive an 80% or 90% level of correctness. This is particularly true of The Compass, or even Embracing Horse, which has a deceptively easy appearance.

Make sure that your posture directs the pressure to the upper thigh, or to the outer side of the body in general, but never to the knees, which would indicate that they are being bent inwards. During practice constantly ask yourself "Am I relaxed enough? Am I loose enough?" The body has to open and close in a very specific manner so as to induce the energy flow. The beginner may experience sore tendons, although this is not a serious problem.

Understand that you will encounter the first signs of difficulty almost immediately with the first posture as you try to maintain the correct alignment. Your thighs will hurt, but you have to try to hold the position. Your body may shake or vibrate. This is the time of maximum benefit and you have to keep your body loose while not giving in to the temptation to quit. How can you convince yourself to continue? One way to ease the stress is to focus your attention on something else. Count, for instance, from one to one thousand. You might try to use some psychology on yourself. Remind yourself that you do not have to continue if you do not want to, that you can stop at any time. Tell yourself that this is voluntary and that it is useful pain that your body is experiencing. Consider a doctor inserting a needle into your arm: it is going to hurt, but is ultimately beneficial. This kind of stress in general is not severe, but is rather a combination of physical and mental discomfort. It is a constructive stress that can be made enjoyable when your mind begins to associate it with the resulting sense of vitality.

When you want to advance yourself more rapidly, you can hold the postures longer and make them proportionally lower. If you do not want to push, don't. I advise beginners not to push themselves at first. I do not believe that excessive pain is a good motivator. I would rather see students do a posture consistently at one level of effort. If you attempt too much at one session, the mind will rebel on a subconscious level during the next session. It is better to build up with a regular schedule. The key to solid, long term results is persistence. Once in a while, after you have developed some stamina, give yourself an extra dose (hardship training). Keep in mind that after hardship training you should have enough rest that night or the next couple of nights to fully recuperate.

Hardship training should be attempted only by advanced students. To the old phrase "no pain, no gain," I would add "correct pain, much gain."

I must emphasize the importance of regular scheduling. It enables you to become mentally prepared to complete the sequence. Set time aside each week according to your ability. Make the appointment with yourself, for yourself. Keep this promise to yourself. Even if you are fatigued you should still do it but cut down the duration. This way it will develop into a habit. Quite often it is only the first few minutes that are less than comfortable. Once the body gets involved, the mind follows.

These exercises are entirely different from Taoist sitting meditation or T'ai Chi Ch'uan practice, both of which require an "empty" mind. You may wish to refer to my book, "T'ai Chi Ch'uan Principles and Practice". Nei Kung training basically involves the physical alignment of the body. A relaxed mind is needed, but no special mental approach is necessary. An occasional check of the posture details is all that is required.

To be outstanding in Nei Kung the key is slow, correct growth. Develop maturity and sophistication before you subject yourself to hardship training. Remind yourself that improvement comes through slight discomfort with gradual progress. Give yourself the necessary time to rest and recuperate. Any who try to reach high levels in a short time will give up at an early stage before they even understand the nature of this system. As with all major endeavors in life, formulate your goal and plan your path to it.

For those students who are also interested in martial arts:

There is a saying in Chinese that if you pursue Ch'uan (fighting technique) without practicing (Nei) Kung, when you reach old age you will have nothing to show for your efforts. This statement underlines the importance of Nei Kung training. Success in the martial arts results from the correct execution of many details. Misunderstandings and shortcuts usually spread faster than truth. Many martial arts students are just learning very superficial forms. Without an understanding of the essence of the Kung Fu system, they tend to pursue the "flowery" or showy aspects and lose sight of the goals of training. Kung Fu training is ultimately for the individual artist and not for an audience. It is for an individual's mental and physical development. It is not intended to be performed like a circus act, although some Kung Fu feats can be astonishing. The greatest reward comes from a sophisticated audience which can appreciate the inner level of achievement involved. It is to these practitioners that I dedicate this book.

Part II—The Exercise

How to Use this Book

Before attempting any of the forms, I suggest a thorough reading of the background chapters in Part I. Underline the sections that do not seem clear. Refer to them and read them again. The extra time you spend will pay off in the long run. There are no short cuts in Nei Kung. If you begin the forms immediately without first understanding what you are trying to accomplish, it will certainly lead to mental and physical frustration. Nei Kung encompasses an interpretation of the body's functioning that is unique. An understanding of the goals and processes involved will provide a measure of psychological protection to counter the inevitable difficulties that will arise. Slow, gradual improvement rather than immediate perfection is our aim. The sooner the student adopts this attitude the better.

Having read the background chapters you should then read the instructions through once in order to get an idea of the extent of the workout procedure. For some, the postures may feel awkward and pointless at first. Nevertheless, seemingly insignificant details in the instructions will have a great bearing on your success or failure. An understanding of the intent behind these details will bind your will to the word.

Once you have read the background chapters and the instructions and have mentally assimilated as much as you can, you will be ready to commence the forms. Beginning with the first form, follow the alignment instructions while positioning yourself. I recommend that you have a full-length mirror on your right or left side to make sure that certain aspects of your posture, such as "tucking in" (see page 23) are correct. Follow the instructions to the last detail, as with a cookbook recipe. Success or failure depends on your habit of practice and your attitude towards it.

Do not be alarmed by certain responses like shaking or vibrating in the limbs, or sweating. These are good signs indicating the beginning of the process of transforming chi energy. Certain other reactions which are potentially hazardous will be addressed individually, form by form. They are caused by incorrect posture and can be harmful if prolonged. Again, caution and gradual progress is the proper way to learn Nei Kung. Beginning students may need more rest and sleep as their bodies become accustomed to this process of energy transformation.

The best time to practice Nei Kung is early in the morning and on an empty stomach. The advantage of the morning is that the body is relaxed and has more stamina to perform the postures. An empty stomach will ensure that the chi is not siphoned off to digestive processes. These conditions are ideal for generating and accumulating chi. The first time that you attempt Nei Kung it is particularly important that you work in the early morning. You will definitely feel the slight beginnings of chi flow and it will continue to some degree for the rest of the day. This should give you the incentive to carry on diligently with the program.

Though early morning is the optimum time for practice, the forms may also be done at mid-day or in the early evening. The time to avoid is just before you prepare for sleep. When your body is tired and your mind is clogged with the events of the day, you will be more likely to make mistakes. The frame of mind needed to "relax into" the postures will not be readily available. If you are able to complete the exercises, you will succeed in charging up the body with chi but may have some difficulty falling asleep. Although you may at first find it complicated to arrange a training schedule, it is important to remind yourself that Nei

Kung is for your benefit. You should set up a time to practice and hold to your program.

During your initial training, perform only one or two new exercises per session. After you have incorporated the entire set of ten forms in sequence, you can use the training program on page 73 as a guideline.

Again I wish to emphasize the importance of thoroughly understanding the elements outlined in the section on the "Basics" as they apply to each exercise.

The Postures:

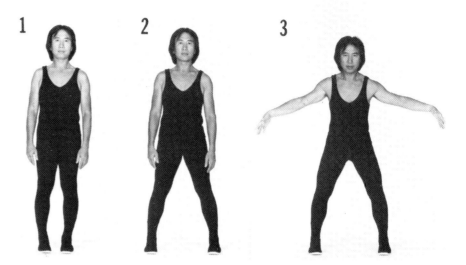

**First Form:
Embracing Horse**

1) Stand upright with the top of the head suspended as if by a string. Let the body sink down with the shoulders lowered. The feet should be parallel and close together. The legs should be straight with the knees almost locked. Distribute the weight equally on each leg. This position is called the neutral stance. Slow the pace of your breathing and gradually deepen each breath. Continue with this relaxed, continuous, deep breathing (see page 26) throughout this exercise. Inhale slowly so that the air will be pushed down expanding the lower abdomen. Exhale in a relaxed way, but let out an extra bit of air at the end. When you feel calm and centered, proceed with the next movement.

2) With the head still suspended, take one step laterally, so that the feet are spaced wider apart than shoulder width and are parallel to each other.

3, 4, 5) Allow the body to sink down by bending the knees and tucking in the pelvis.

Turn the toes in slightly and spread the knees apart, focusing most of the body weight on the heels and outer edges of the feet. The weight should be distributed equally on each leg throughout this exercise. Simultaneously raise both arms up and forward in a slight arc from behind until they form a circle in front of you with your hands, arms, shoulders, and chest forming a smooth curve, as if encircling a sphere. The palms should face the chest with the fingers slightly stretched. Be sure that the shoulders and the elbows are lowered and that the pelvis is tucked in (see page 23 for a detailed explanation).

Maintain this position while remembering to hold the head as if suspended from above. You can lean the torso slightly forward for easier positioning as long as the back is kept straight. Later you can "rock back" to a more vertical posture, as in the side view. You should sense your body pressing down on the floor with most of the weight felt in the heels and outer edges of the feet. The legs should be

4   **5**

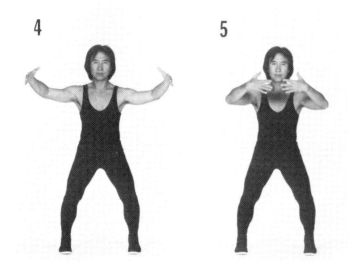

somewhat bow-shaped to facilitate this weight distribution. If the form is done properly, you should feel pressure on the outside of the thighs. Make sure that no stress is felt on the knees.

Initially, this position should be held for three minutes while maintaining relaxation and deep breathing. Breathe with the diaphragm, through the nose, and as silently as possible. The mouth should be closed with the teeth gently meshed together. The front upper surface of the tongue should rest on the roof of the mouth, just behind the front teeth. Gaze at a point directly ahead through relaxed eyelids. The mind is calm and meditative. Gradually, the duration of this form can be increased to 15 minutes.

The three key points of this form are the suspension of the head (see page 22), the tucking in of the pelvis (see page 23), and the relaxation of the body. The stress should be on the outside of the thighs, not on the knees.

Caution: if there is stress on the knees, immediately recheck your alignment, making sure that you have the knees out and the toes in. Your sense of suspending the head and letting the body sink down will aid you in increasing the duration of this exercise. However, you should always have some feeling of discomfort in the thighs, especially toward the end of this form. Avoid the tendency to fidget. Adjust your posture with calm, controlled movements. When you develop to the point where you do not feel this discomfort, make your stance wider and sink down lower accordingly.

This form, which is paramount in this series, is designed to align the meridians of the body and to open the channels in order to stimulate the flow of chi. When performed correctly, chi will be generated continuously. A feeling of vibration in the body is a sign of progress with this posture. When this first form is completed, resume the neutral position and lightly shake each leg.

5

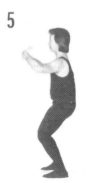

side view

37

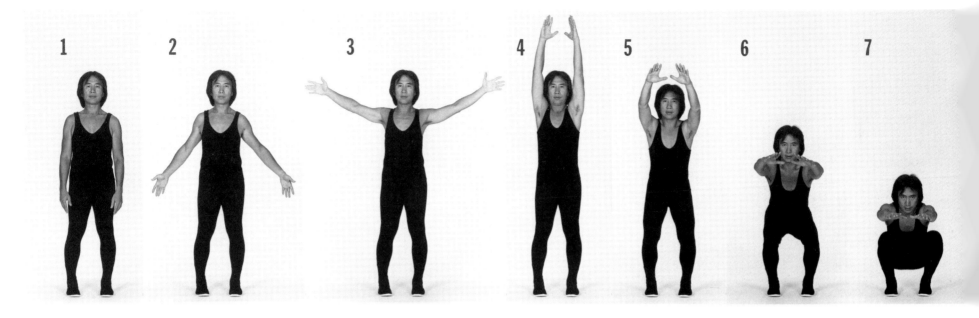

Second Form:
Riding the Wild Horse,
middle stance

1) Stand in the neutral position with the feet placed parallel and spaced narrower than the shoulder width. Turn the toes in slightly and spread the knees apart, focusing most of the body weight on the heels and outer edges of the feet. The weight should be distributed equally on each leg throughout this exercise.

2, 3) With the head still suspended, inhale slowly and deeply from the diaphragm while pulling the arms backward and raising them upward in a slow circular motion, stretching them as far as possible so as to open the shoulder joints.

4) Stop when the arms are parallel overhead. Complete the inhalation simultaneously. The hands should not touch each other. The arms and fingers should stretch upward as if being pulled from above by the finger tips.

5, 6, 7) Exhale slowly, tuck in the pelvis, and bend the knees as you slowly sink down. It is important to maintain the tucked in position of the pelvis throughout this exercise. Extend the arms and hands outward in front of you as far as possible as you settle into a squatting position with the knees spread apart. Hold this lowest position for up to five seconds as you continue to slowly complete the exhalation. Lower the body only as far as possible without discomfort. The arms and fingers should stretch forward. Maintain the tucked in position of the pelvis. The legs should be somewhat bowed with most of the weight on the heels and the outer edges of the feet. Refer to the side views for correct positioning.

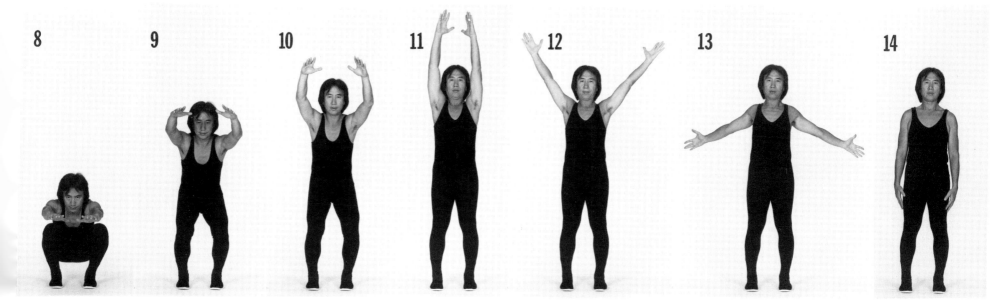

8, 9, 10, 11) Inhale slowly, keeping the pelvis tucked in, and push down on the heels to raise the body up. Extending the arms as far as possible in front of the body, raise them up gradually until you are standing and they are parallel overhead. Complete the inhalation when the arms stop.

12, 13) Exhale slowly as you lower the arms back and downward in a slow circular motion, stretching them out and back as much as possible, until they are at your sides. The shoulders should be relaxed and kept lowered as the arms are stretched back. Complete the exhalation as your arms reach your sides.

14) From this starting position, repeat the form one to five times. The duration from the beginning to the squatting position should take 15 to 20 seconds and the reversal should be about the same.

The additional emphasis on tucking in the pelvis for this exercise assures that the knees can be spread apart. Otherwise, improper stress on the knees can result in injury. Many avoid the traditional "deep knee bends" of calisthenics due to a misunderstanding of the correct technique described here.

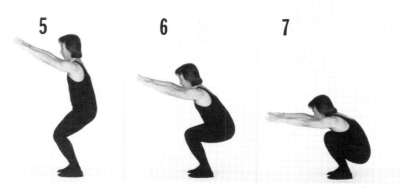

side view

39

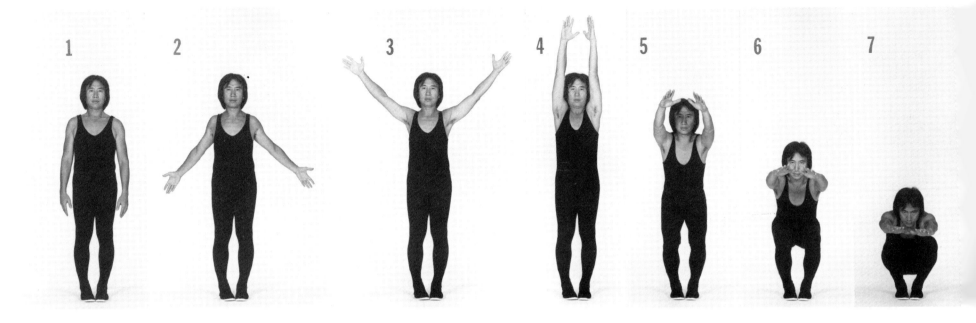

**Second Form:
Riding the Wild Horse,
small stance**

1) Stand in the neutral position with the feet placed so that the toes touch each other while the heels are separated by several inches. Make sure the knees do not touch. If this cannot be avoided because of the way you are built, open the heels until the knees separate, and make sure that the knees do not touch each other during the movement. Most of the body weight will be concentrated on the heels and outer edges of the feet. The weight should be distributed equally on each leg throughout this exercise.

2, 3) With the head still suspended, inhale slowly and deeply from the diaphragm while pulling the arms backward and raising them upward in a slow circular motion, stretching them as far as possible so as to open the shoulder joints.

4) Stop when the arms are parallel overhead. Complete the inhalation simultaneously.

The hands should not touch each other. The arms and fingers should stretch upward as if being pulled from above by the finger tips.

5, 6, 7) Exhale slowly, tuck in the pelvis, and bend the knees as you slowly sink down. It is important to maintain the tucked in position of the pelvis throughout this exercise. Extend the arms and hands outward in front of you as far as possible as you settle into a squatting position with the knees spread apart. Hold this lowest position for up to five seconds as you continue to slowly complete the exhalation. Lower the body only as far as possible without discomfort. The arms and fingers should stretch forward. Maintain the tucked in position of the pelvis. The legs should be somewhat bowed with most of the weight on the heels and outer edges of the feet. Refer to the side views for correct positioning.

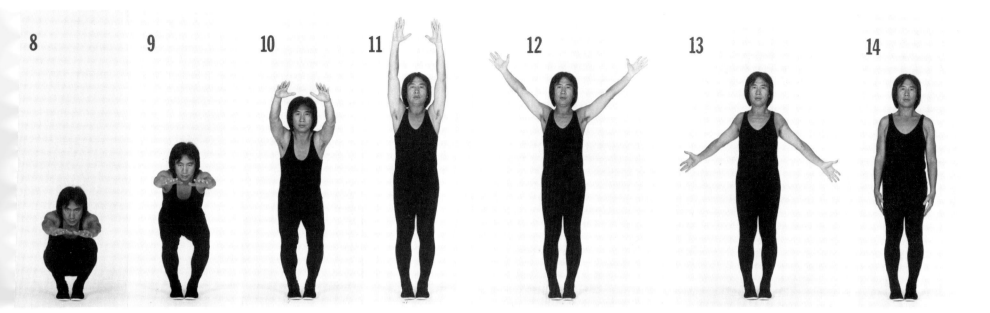

8, 9, 10, 11) Inhale slowly, keeping the pelvis tucked in, and push down on the heels to raise the body up. Extending the arms as far as possible in front of the body, raise them up gradually until you are standing and they are parallel overhead. Complete the inhalation when the arms stop.

12, 13) Exhale slowly as you lower the arms back and downward in a slow circular motion, stretching them out and back as much as possible, until they are at your sides. The shoulders should be relaxed and kept lowered as the arms are stretched back. Complete the exhalation as your arms reach your sides.

14) From this starting position, repeat the form one to five times. The duration from the beginning to the squatting position should take 15 to 20 seconds and the reversal should be about the same.

The additional emphasis on tucking in the pelvis for this exercise assures that the knees can be spread apart. Otherwise, improper stress on the knees can result in injury. Many avoid the traditional "deep knee bends" of calisthenics due to a misunderstanding of the correct technique described here.

5 6 7

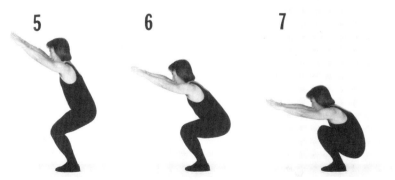

side view

41

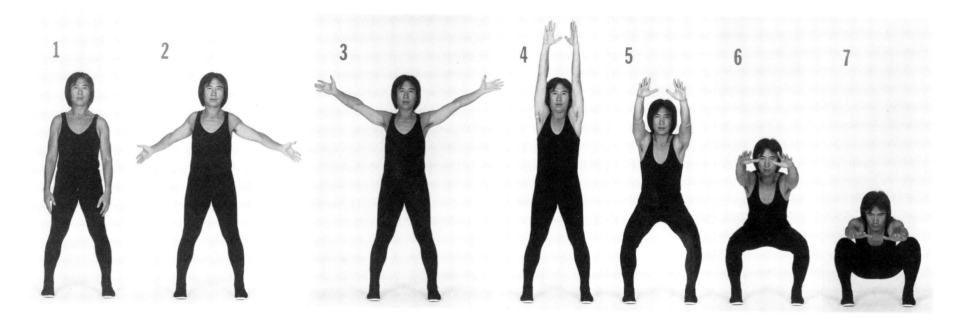

**Second Form:
Riding the Wild Horse,
large stance**

1) Stand in the neutral position with the feet spaced wider apart than the shoulder width. Turn the toes in slightly and spread the knees apart, focusing most of the body weight on the heels and outer edges of the feet. The weight should be distributed equally on each leg throughout this exercise.

2, 3) With the head still suspended, inhale slowly and deeply from the diaphragm while pulling the arms backward and raising them upward in a slow circular motion, stretching them as far as possible so as to open the shoulder joints.

4) Stop when the arms are parallel overhead. Complete the inhalation simultaneously. The hands should not touch each other. The arms and fingers should stretch upward as if being pulled from above by the finger tips.

5, 6, 7) Exhale slowly, tuck in the pelvis, and bend the knees as you slowly sink down. It is important to maintain the tucked in position of the pelvis throughout this exercise. Extend the arms and hands outward in front of you as far as possible as you settle into a squatting position with the knees spread apart. Hold this lowest position for up to five seconds as you continue to slowly complete the exhalation. Lower the body only as far as possible without discomfort. The arms and fingers should stretch forward. Maintain the tucked in position of the pelvis. The legs should be somewhat bowed with most of the weight on the heels and outer edges of the feet. Refer to the side views for correct positioning.

8, 9, 10, 11) Inhale slowly, keeping the pelvis tucked in, and push down on the heels to

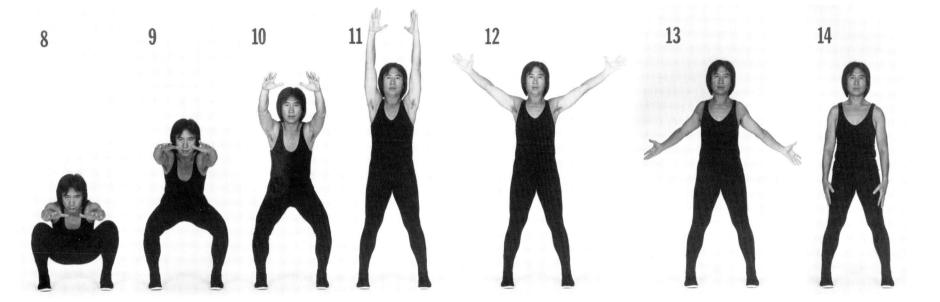

8   9   10   11   12   13   14

raise the body up. Extending the arms as far as possible in front of the body, raise them up gradually until you are standing and they are parallel overhead. Complete the inhalation when the arms stop.

12, 13) Exhale slowly as you lower the arms back and downward in a slow circular motion, stretching them out and back as much as possible, until they are at your sides. The shoulders should be relaxed and kept lowered as the arms are stretched back. Complete the exhalation as your arms reach your sides.

14) From this starting position, repeat the form one to five times. The duration from the beginning to the squatting position should take 15 to 20 seconds and the reversal should be about the same.

The additional emphasis on tucking in the pelvis for this exercise assures that the knees can be spread apart. Otherwise, improper stress on the knees can result in injury. Many avoid the traditional "deep knee bends" of calisthenics due to a misunderstanding of the correct technique described here.

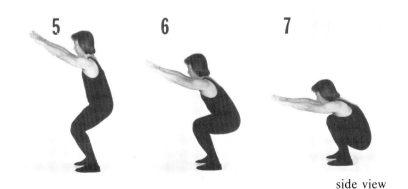

5   6   7

side view

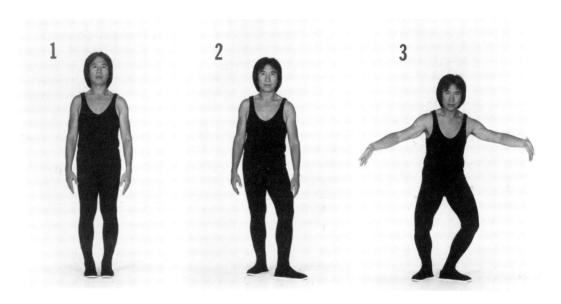

**Third Form:
Playing P'i P'a,*
right side**

1, 2) From the neutral stance, step forward with the left foot being particularly careful to place it at a 60 degree angle to the front-back axis of the body. Use relaxed, continuous, deep breathing throughout this exercise.

3, 4) Bend both knees and open the arms, bringing them from the back to the front as you bring your right leg forward. Your balance should be maintained on your left leg. The upper torso and arms should form a smoothly rounded shape as the right foot comes to rest on its heel. With your left palm facing your right elbow, the fingers should be slightly stretched and pointed upward.

5) Most of the weight of the body (about 90%) will be carried by the left leg, and it will be concentrated on the heel and outer edge of the left foot. The pelvis should be kept tucked in. Hold this position for one-half to three minutes. If done correctly, stress will be felt on

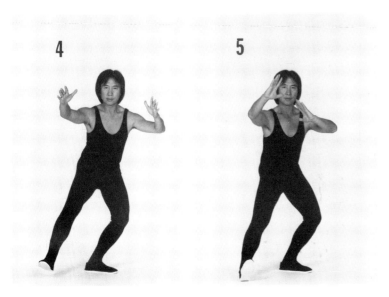

the outer portion of the thigh of the left leg. *Caution:* Make sure that there is no stress felt on the knee. If so, adjust the left knee so that it is over the toes of the left foot. The body weight should be concentrated on the heel and outer edge of the left foot, which is kept at a 60 degree angle to the front-back axis of the body.

Do not force this posture if it is too stressful. If you are tired, relax, check your suspension (see page 22) and the tension will ease. Avoid fidgeting. Adjust the posture with calm, controlled movements. As with Embracing Horse, a feeling of vibration is a sign of progress with this exercise.

---

*The P'i P'a is a traditional Chinese stringed instrument.

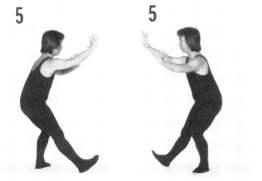

side view

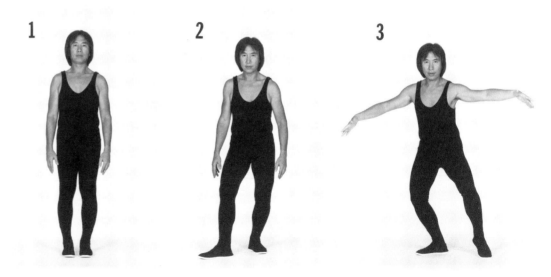

**Third Form:
Playing P'i P'a,
left side**

1, 2) From the neutral stance, step forward with the right foot being particularly careful to place it at a 60 degree angle to the front-back axis of the body. Use relaxed, continuous, deep breathing throughout this exercise.

3, 4) Bend both knees and open the arms, bringing them from the back to the front as you bring your left leg forward. Your balance should be maintained on your right leg. The upper torso and arms should form a smoothly rounded shape as the left foot comes to rest on its heel. With your right palm facing your left elbow, the fingers should be slightly stretched and pointed upward.

5) Most of the weight of the body (about 90%) will be carried by the right leg, and it will be concentrated on the heel and outer edge of the right foot. The pelvis should be kept tucked in. Hold this position for one-half

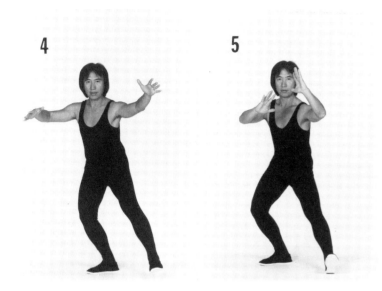

4 **5**

to three minutes. If done correctly, stress will be felt on the outer portion of the thigh of the right leg. *Caution:* Make sure that there is no stress felt on the knee. If so, adjust the right knee so that it is over the toes of the right foot. The body weight should be concentrated on the heel and outer edge of the right foot, which is kept at a 60 degree angle to the front-back axis of the body.

Do not force this posture if it is too stressful. If you are tired, relax, check your suspension (see page 22) and the tension will ease. Avoid fidgeting. Adjust the posture with calm, controlled movements. As with Embracing Horse, a feeling of vibration is a sign of progress with this exercise.

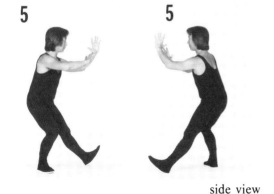

5 **5**

side view

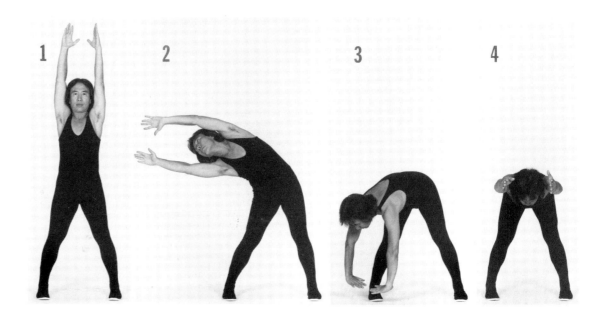

**Fourth Form:
The Compass,
right side**

1) Stand in the neutral position with the feet parallel and wider apart than the shoulder width. Your breathing should be relaxed, continuous, and deep throughout this sequence. Turn the toes in slightly and spread the knees apart, focusing most of the body weight on the heels and outer edges of the feet. Distribute the weight equally on each leg. Slowly pull the arms backward and raise them upward until they point overhead. The arms and fingers should stretch out, as if they are being pulled from above.

2) Slowly drop to the right at the waist, keeping the pelvis facing forward, and relaxing the whole body so that gravity pulls the upper torso to its limit. Hold this position for 10 to 15 seconds. Note that the body is kept within a vertical plane. The arms and fingers stretch out straight. The body weight shifts slightly to the right leg.

3) Slowly roll the waist a few degrees forward, allowing gravity to pull the torso down, bringing the arms into a position close to the right leg. You should feel a stretching on the back of this leg as you hold this position for 15 to 20 seconds. Do not bend the knees. The arms and hands should form a spherical shape as the fingers stretch toward each other with the palms facing down. However, the hands should not touch each other or the ground.

4) Roll the waist forward, keeping the back flat and the arms parallel in front of the torso. Hold for 20 seconds. *Caution:* do not arch the back. Breathe deeply; do not hold your breath. Do not let the head or arms droop down. Keep the shoulders up. View yourself in a mirror to see if your back is flat, as in the side view. Distribute the weight equally on each leg.

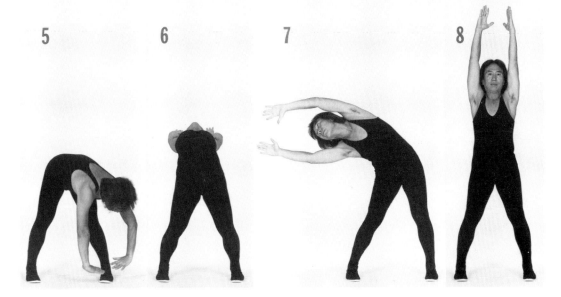

5) Roll to the left, letting the arms and torso drop close to the left leg. You should feel a stretching on the back of the left leg. Again, the fingers point toward each other with the palms facing down. Hold this position for 15 to 20 seconds. The weight is now slightly more on the left leg.

6) Roll the torso leftward and to the back without raising it up, keeping the arms parallel with the head. The knees and legs can bend back slightly, as in the side view. Let the head drop gently with the pull of gravity. Distribute the weight equally on each leg.

7, 8) Roll the torso to the right, stretching the arms and fingers, and shifting the weight to the right leg. After holding this position briefly, raise the torso and the arms to the starting position.

This sequence can be repeated up to three more times, starting from position 2. Keep in mind that the rolling of the torso lets gravity do the work of continuously stretching the legs, waist, and arms. Make sure the toes stay pointed slightly inward throughout this movement.

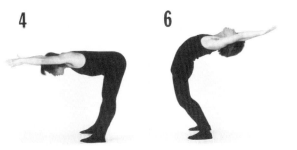

side view

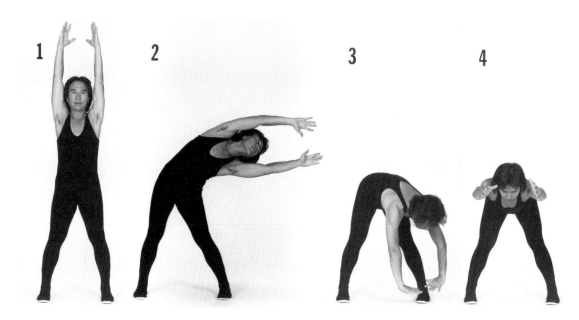

**Fourth Form:
The Compass,
left side**

1) Stand in the neutral position with the feet parallel and wider apart than the shoulder width. Your breathing should be relaxed, continuous, and deep throughout this sequence. Turn the toes in slightly and spread the knees apart, focusing most of the body weight on the heels and outer edges of the feet. Distribute the weight equally on each leg. Slowly pull the arms backward and raise them upward until they point overhead. The arms and fingers should stretch out, as if they are being pulled from above.

2) Slowly drop to the left at the waist, keeping the pelvis facing forward, and relaxing the whole body so that gravity pulls the upper torso to its limit. Hold this position for 10 to 15 seconds. Note that the body is kept within a vertical plane. The arms and fingers stretch out straight. The body weight shifts slightly to the left leg.

3) Slowly roll the waist a few degrees forward, allowing gravity to pull the torso down, bringing the arms into a position close to the left leg. You should feel a stretching on the back of this leg as you hold this position for 15 to 20 seconds. Do not bend the knees. The arms and hands should form a spherical shape as the fingers stretch toward each other with the palms facing down. However, the hands should not touch each other or the ground.

4) Roll the waist forward, keeping the back flat and the arms parallel in front of the torso. Hold for 20 seconds. *Caution:* do not arch the back. Breathe deeply; do not hold your breath. Do not let the head or arms droop down. Keep the shoulders up. View yourself in a mirror to see if your back is flat, as in the side view. Distribute the weight equally on each leg.

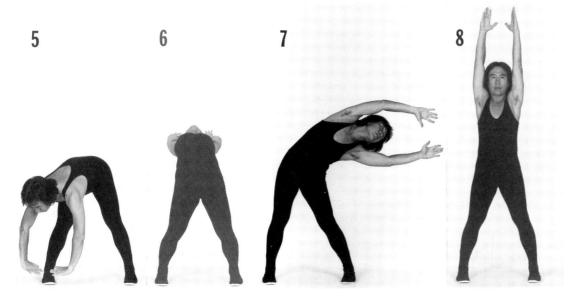

5) Roll to the right, letting the arms and torso drop close to the right leg. You should feel a stretching on the back of the right leg. Again, the fingers point toward each other with the palms facing down. Hold this position for 15 to 20 seconds. The weight is now slightly more on the right leg.

6) Roll the torso rightward and to the back without raising it up, keeping the arms parallel with the head. The knees and legs can bend back slightly, as in the side view. Let the head drop gently with the pull of gravity. Distribute the weight equally on each leg.

7, 8) Roll the torso to the left, stretching the arms and fingers, and shifting the weight to the left leg. After holding this position briefly, raise the torso and the arms to the starting position.

This sequence can be repeated up to three more times, starting from position 2. Keep in mind that the rolling of the torso lets gravity do the work of continuously stretching the legs, waist, and arms. Make sure the toes stay pointed slightly inward throughout this movement.

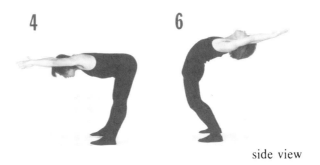

side view

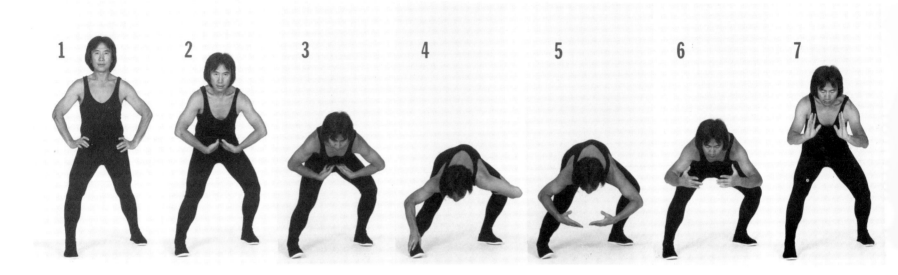

Fifth Form:
Double Dragons Leap from Sea, right side

1) Stand with the feet positioned as in the photograph and with the hands on the hips. The right leg should be forward with the knee over the toe, the left leg back and almost, but not quite, locked straight. This positioning is commonly called the "Bow and Arrow Stance." The weight distribution should be about 70% on the front foot and 30% on the back foot, concentrated on the heels and outer edges of the feet. Maintain a tucked in pelvis. Your breathing should be relaxed, continuous, and deep.

2, 3) Locating a point about two inches below the navel, push the body backward with your fingers, gradually shifting the weight toward the back leg as you bend the torso forward and downward. Exhale deeply while sinking back. Continue with the deep breathing.

4) Place the left hand on the left knee, and gently push it outward and backward to line up the knee on top of the toes. *Caution:* Bending the knee inward toward the center of

the body can be harmful. About 70% of the body weight should now be carried by the left leg with the pelvis properly tucked in. However, avoid the tendency to shift the pelvis laterally toward the left. The pelvis should be centered between the feet throughout this exercise, whether in the forward or rearward position. Grasp the right ankle with the right hand, and slowly stretch the tendons along the back of the right leg by bending the torso forward and downward. The weight of the body should still be felt on the heels and outer edges of the feet. Hold this position for 20 seconds.

5, 6) With the chest concave, arms held in a rounded shape, and the fingers slightly stretched, slowly push forward off the heel of the back leg. Inhale deeply while you shift forward. Maintain a tucked in pelvis. Refer also to the side views.

7, 8) Continue shifting forward until the right knee is over the toe and the left leg is almost straight with the rounded arms and

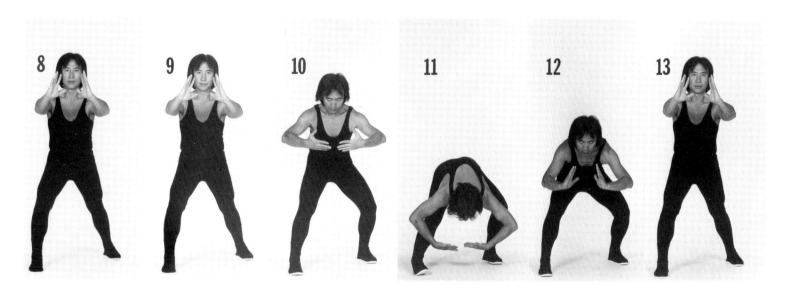

hands extending as you complete your inhalation. The fingers should also be slightly stretched. Continue with relaxed, natural breathing. Hold this position for five to ten seconds.

9, 10, 11) Slowly shift the pelvis backward, while bending the torso forward and downward, until about 70% of the weight is on the rear left leg. Again, try to fold the body below the navel. Simultaneously, rotate the palms inward until they face upward. The arms and hands should be rounded with the fingers slightly stretched. Exhale during this movement and continue exhaling as you maintain the last position for up to five seconds.

12, 13) Inhale as you slowly push upward and forward off the back leg, rotating the palms of both hands outward. The rounded arms and hands should extend forward as you complete your inhalation. Again, the right knee ends up over the toes and the left leg is almost straight.

Repeat 9, 10, 11, 12, 13 up to four more times slowly. Use one deep exhalation for each sink-back and one deep inhalation for each push-forward.

Advanced students can then repeat 9, 10, 11, 12, 13 up to ten times as rapidly as possible, with one quick, deep exhalation for each sink-back and one quick, deep inhalation for each push-forward. Refer to item 8 of the "Basics" section for more information about the breathing (see page 26).

Note that throughout this exercise the hips should face forward, parallel to the ground, and should be centered between the feet. Remember to keep the pelvis tucked in throughout. When performed properly, the push should feel solid and powerful, as it employs the entire body in an integrated propulsion. There will be a continuous linkage from the heels to the fingertips.

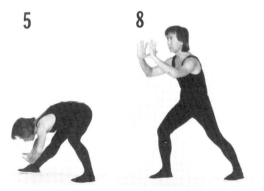

side view   diagonal view

53

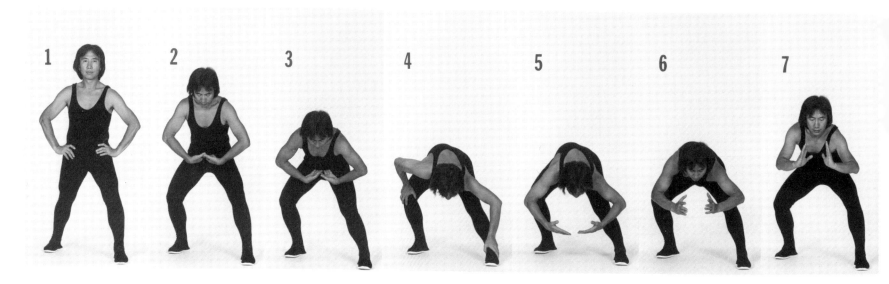

**Fifth Form:
Double Dragons Leap from Sea,
left side**

1) Stand with the feet positioned as in the photograph and with the hands on the hips. The left leg should be forward with the knee over the toe, the right leg back and almost, but not quite, locked straight. This positioning is commonly called the "Bow and Arrow Stance." The weight distribution should be about 70% on the front foot and 30% on the back foot, concentrated on the heels and outer edges of the feet. Maintain a tucked in pelvis. Your breathing should be relaxed, continuous, and deep.

2, 3) Locating a point about two inches below the navel, push the body backward with your fingers, gradually shifting the weight toward the back leg as you bend the torso forward and downward. Exhale deeply while sinking back. Continue with the deep breathing.

4) Place the right hand on the right knee, and gently push it outward and backward to line up the knee on top of the toes. *Caution:* Bending the knee inward toward the center of

the body can be harmful. About 70% of the body weight should now be carried by the right leg with the pelvis properly tucked in. However, avoid the tendency to shift the pelvis laterally toward the right. The pelvis should be centered between the feet throughout this exercise, whether in the forward or rearward position. Grasp the left ankle with the left hand, and slowly stretch the tendons along the back of the left leg by bending the torso forward and downward. The weight of the body should still be felt on the heels and outer edges of the feet. Hold this position for 20 seconds.

5, 6) With the chest concave, arms held in a rounded shape, and the fingers slightly stretched, slowly push forward off the heel of the back leg. Inhale deeply while you shift forward. Maintain a tucked in pelvis. Refer also to the side views.

7, 8) Continue shifting forward until the left knee is over the toe and the right leg is almost straight with the rounded arms and hands extending as you complete your inhala-

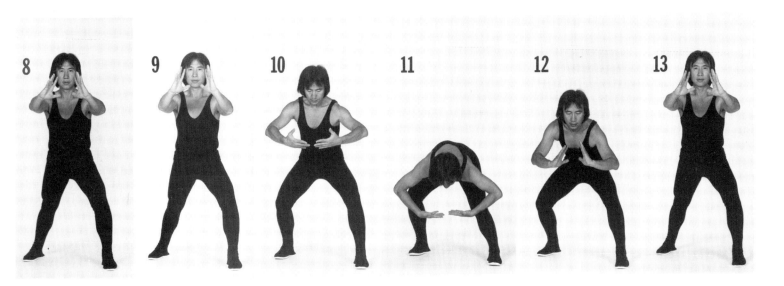

tion. The fingers should also be slightly stretched. Continue with relaxed, natural breathing. Hold this position for five to ten seconds.

9, 10, 11) Slowly shift the pelvis backward, while bending the torso forward and downward, until about 70% of the weight is on the rear right leg. Again, try to "fold" the body below the navel. Simultaneously, rotate the palms inward until they face upward. The arms and hands should be rounded with the fingers slightly stretched. Exhale during this movement and continue exhaling as you maintain the last position for up to five seconds.

12, 13) Inhale as you slowly push upward and forward off the back leg, rotating the palms of both hands outward. The rounded arms and hands should extend forward as you complete your inhalation. Again, the left knee ends up over the toes and the right leg is almost straight.

Repeat 9, 10, 11, 12, 13 up to four more times slowly. Use one deep exhalation for each sink-back and one deep inhalation for each push-forward.

Advanced students can then repeat 9, 10, 11, 12, 13 up to 10 times as rapidly as possible, with one quick, deep exhalation for each sink-back and one quick, deep inhalation for each push-forward. Refer to item 8 of the "Basics" section for more information about the breathing (see page 26).

Note that throughout this exercise the hips should face forward, parallel to the ground, and should be centered between the feet. Remember to keep the pelvis tucked in throughout. When performed properly, the push should feel solid and powerful, as it employs the entire body in an integrated propulsion. There will be a continuous linkage from the heels to the fingertips.

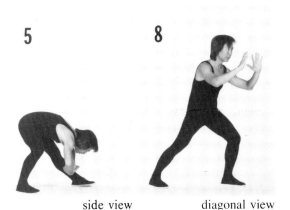

side view   diagonal view

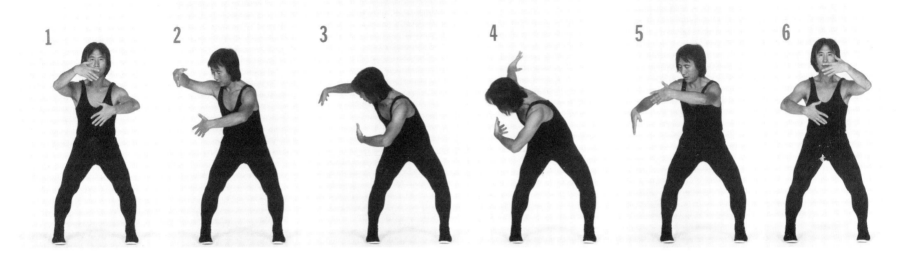

Sixth Form:
Rhinoceros Gazes at the Moon

1) Stand in the neutral position with the feet parallel and wider apart than the shoulder width. The weight should be distributed equally on each leg throughout this exercise. Let the body sink down by bending the knees and tucking in the pelvis. Turn the toes in slightly and spread the knees apart, focusing most of the weight on the heels and outer edges of the feet. Extend the arms in front of the torso in a rounded shape with the chest concave, as if encircling a sphere. Place the right hand above the left with the palms facing the body. The breathing should be relaxed, continuous, and deep throughout this exercise.

2, 3) Slowly rotate the upper torso to the right, keeping the hips in a forward-facing position while sweeping the arms to the rear and twisting the palms upward. The upper body should be rounded as it twists at the waist. The hips and legs should remain fixed throughout this movement.

4) When you can rotate the torso no farther, continue to slowly sweep the right arm backward, still twisting the palms upward. Keep the left arm in a rounded shape so that you feel the connection between the two hands through the upper torso, as if all were one solid piece united by the line of tendons along the arms. Maintain a continuous tension of the waist and torso at the point of maximum twisting. Try to breathe continuously. Do not hold your breath. Hold this position for eight to ten seconds.

5, 6) Rotate the upper torso back to the front with the left hand positioned above the right hand.

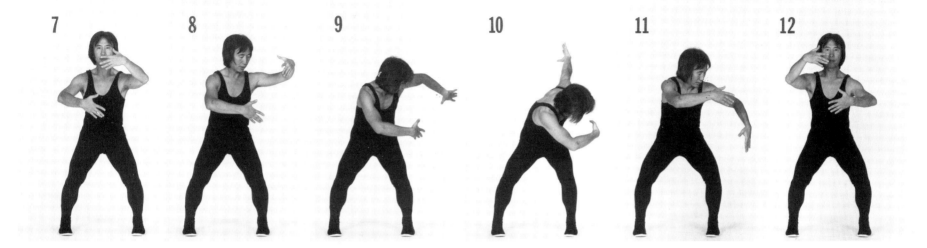

7, 8, 9) Continue the rotation to the left side, slowly sweeping the left arm to the back and twisting the palms upward. The right arm should be smoothly rounded. It should not collapse into the body.

10) Hold this position for 8 to 10 seconds. Again, maintain a stretching twist while breathing continuously. Refer also to the side view.

11, 12) Slowly rotate the upper torso back toward the right in a continuous movement.

Repeat the sequence one to five more times. The important points of this stance are tucking in the pelvis, turning the toes in and positioning the knees over the toes. Maintaining roundness of the arms through the upper body and the continuous tension at the point of maximum twisting are the specific goals of this exercise.

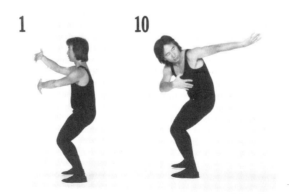

side view

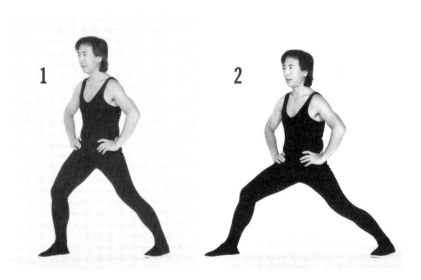

**Seventh Form:
Riding Tiger,
right side**

1) Tuck in the pelvis, place the hands on the hips, and position the feet as in the photograph. There should be slightly more weight on the right leg. Open the legs, sliding the right foot forward along a straight line emanating from the center of the body, while sliding the left leg backward along the same line. Try to keep the feet parallel and at a 45 degree angle to this line as you continue. Breathing should be relaxed, continuous, and deep during this exercise.

2, 3) Slowly open the legs wider, keeping the knees slightly bent as you drop down a few inches at a time and hold each position for a few seconds. The feet should be flat on the ground and there should be slightly more weight on the right foot. The tucked in pelvis should face in the same 45 degree direction as the right foot, while the torso should twist a bit more to the right.

58

3   **4**

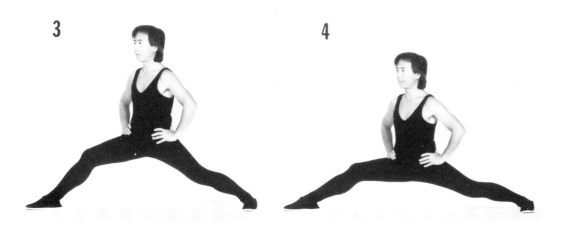

4) Stretch the legs as far apart as possible and hold the final position for about eight seconds. The feet will no longer be exactly parallel, but the toes should be pointed inward as much as possible, with both knees bent and the feet flat. The purpose is not just to go as low as possible, but to hold your lowest position while maintaining the key details: a relaxed body with a tucked in pelvis, bent knees, the feet flat on the ground, and the weight on the heels and outer edges of the feet.

Return to the starting position by drawing up the front foot a few inches at a time. This posture can be repeated one or two more times, alternating with "Riding Tiger, left side."

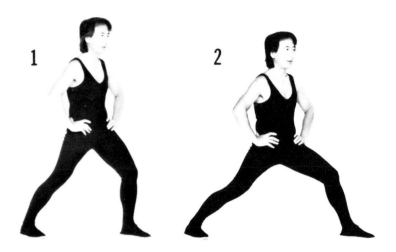

**Seventh Form:
Riding Tiger,
left side**

1) Tuck in the pelvis, place the hands on the hips, and position the feet as in the photograph. There should be slightly more weight on the left leg. Open the legs, sliding the left foot forward along a straight line emanating from the center of the body, while sliding the right leg backward along the same line. Try to keep the feet parallel and at a 45 degree angle to this line as you continue. Breathing should be relaxed, continuous, and deep during this exercise.

2, 3) Slowly open the legs wider, keeping the knees slightly bent as you drop down a few inches at a time and hold each position for a few seconds. The feet should be flat on the ground and there should be slightly more weight on the left foot. The tucked in pelvis should face in the same 45 degree direction as the left foot, while the torso should twist a bit more to the left.

3   **4**

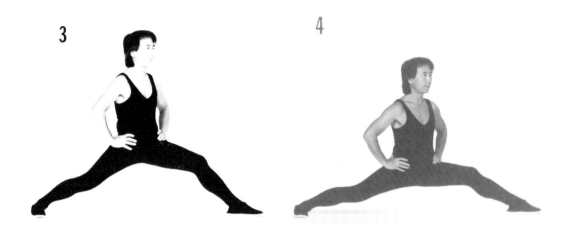

4) Stretch the legs as far apart as possible and hold the final position for about eight seconds. The feet will no longer be exactly parallel, but the toes should be pointed inward as much as possible, with both knees bent and the feet flat. The purpose is not just to go as low as possible, but to hold your lowest position while maintaining the key details: a relaxed body with a tucked in pelvis, bent knees, the feet flat on the ground, and the weight on the heels and outer edges of the feet.

Return to the starting position by drawing up the front foot a few inches at a time. This posture can be repeated one or two more times, alternating with "Riding Tiger, right side."

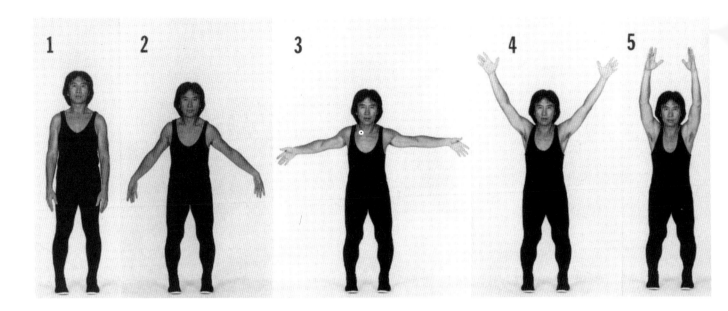

**Eighth Form:
Phoenix Spreads Wings,
forward**

1) Stand in the neutral position with both feet parallel and narrower than the shoulder width. Let the body sink down by bending the knees and tucking in the pelvis. Turn the toes in slightly and spread the knees apart, focusing most of the body weight on the heels and outer edges of the feet. The weight should be distributed equally on each leg throughout this exercise. Lean the torso forward slightly. The breathing should be relaxed, continuous, and deep during this movement.

2, 3, 4, 5, 6, 7, 8) Continuously swing the arms up from behind and then down to the front by using a slight pumping motion of the lower torso. Do not control the arms from the shoulders; rather, use the centrifugal force emanating from the pumping motion of the lower torso. Allow the shoulders to be opened to the maximum extent. When the torso rises up, the arms follow; when the torso drops, the arms follow. The hands should repeatedly trace an oval path. The swinging arms pivot at

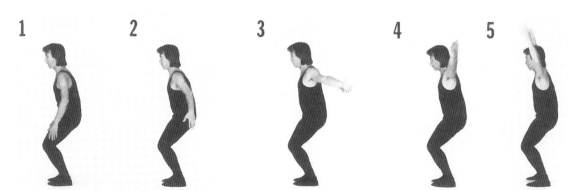

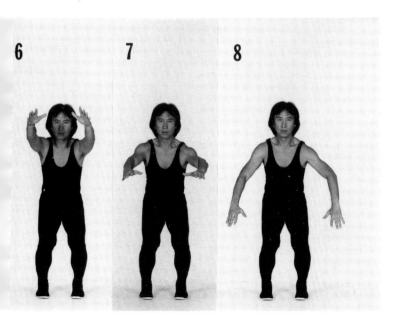

the shoulder joint but, again, are not controlled from this point. The knees should be bent throughout to absorb some of the motion. Do not straighten the legs. Remember to maintain a concave chest. The pelvis is kept tucked in, the knees are out, the toes are in, and the weight is mostly on the heels and outer edges of the feet.

The hands should swing as high as possible, but without touching each other. The joints should be as loose as possible. The arms should feel so relaxed that they do not seem to be part of the body. *Caution:* Forceful, unrestrained swinging may pull a muscle or tendon, so stay loose.

In the beginning, execute this movement for 30 to 50 continuous rotations of the arms at a moderate speed. As you become more proficient, add another 10 to 20 continuous rotations at a higher speed.

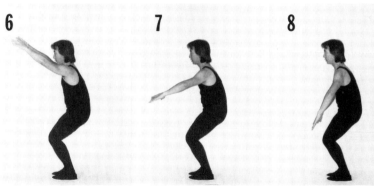

side view

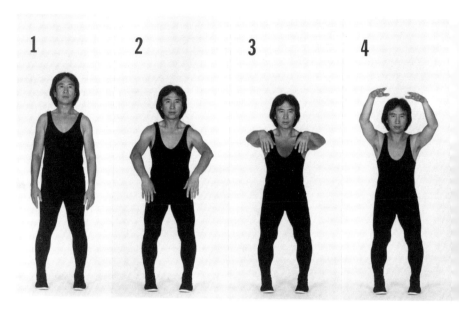

**Eighth Form:
Phoenix Spreads Wings,
backward**

1) Stand in the neutral position with both feet parallel and narrower than the shoulder width. Let the body sink down by bending the knees and tucking in the pelvis. Turn the toes in slightly and spread the knees apart, focusing most of the body weight on the heels and outer edges of the feet. The weight should be distributed equally on each leg throughout this exercise. Lean the torso forward slightly. The breathing should be relaxed, continuous, and deep during this movement.

2, 3, 4, 5, 6, 7, 8) Continuously swing the arms up from the front, then down to the rear by using a slight pumping of the lower torso. Do not control the arms from the shoulders; rather, use the centrifugal force emanating from the pumping motion of the lower torso. Allow the shoulders to be opened to the maximum extent. When the torso rises up, the arms follow; when the torso drops, the arms follow. The hands should repeatedly trace an oval path. The swinging arms pivot at the shoulder

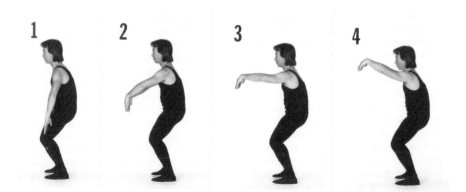

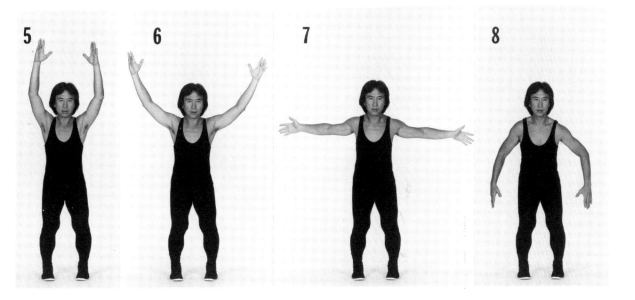

joint but, again, are not controlled from this point. The knees should be bent throughout to absorb some of the motion. Do not straighten the legs. Remember to maintain a concave chest. The pelvis is kept tucked in, the knees are out, the toes are in, and the weight is mostly on the heels and outer edges of the feet.

The hands should swing as high as possible, but without touching each other. The joints should be as loose as possible. The arms should feel so relaxed that they do not seem to be part of the body. *Caution:* Forceful, unrestrained swinging may pull a muscle or tendon, so stay loose.

In the beginning, execute this movement for 30 to 50 continuous rotations of the arms at a moderate speed. As you become more proficient, add another 10 to 20 continuous rotations at a higher speed.

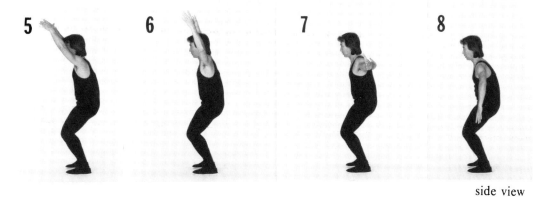

side view

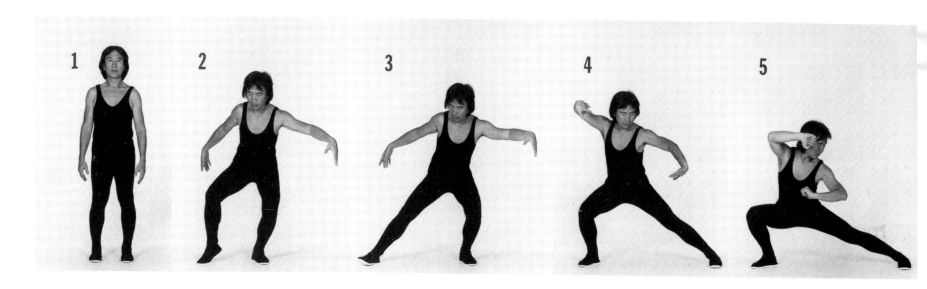

**Ninth Form:
Hitting the Tiger,
right side**

1) Stand in the neutral position with the feet parallel and narrower than the shoulder width. Breathing should be relaxed, continuous, and deep.

2) Begin to inhale a slow, deep breath. Tuck in the pelvis and shift the weight momentarily to the left leg. While turning the torso towards the right, step sideward with the right foot and bring the arms from the back to the front in a circular motion by using a contracting movement of the chest.

3, 4) With one fluid motion shift the weight again, this time to the right leg. Let the hips slowly sink down on the right leg and twist the upper torso towards the left. Continue to inhale the same breath.

5, 6) Loosely clench the fists as you bring the right arm up in an arc to the forehead and the left one in an arc to waist level. The rounded arms and the concave chest should form a smooth curve. Continue to sink down with the upper torso twisting toward the straightened left leg as you lean slightly forward. The left foot can slide outward as you sink down. Make sure the weight of the body is felt on the heel and outer edge of the right foot while taking care to align the right knee over the toes. It is important that this knee does not bend inward. The left foot should be resting flat on the ground, but carrying very little of the body's weight. The entire sinking down motion is rapid, about two to three seconds, and consists of a single inhalation.

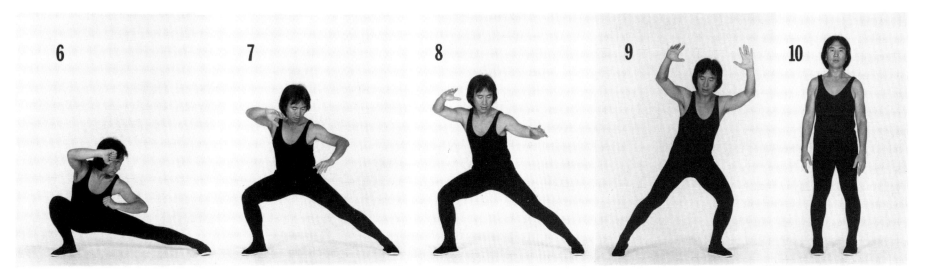

Make sure that the pelvis is still tucked in. Refer also to the side view and the diagonal view for the lowest position.

7, 8, 9, 10) In one fluid motion, return to the original position by pushing off the floor on the heel of the right foot, and reversing the previous arc of the arms. Again, make sure to keep the pelvis tucked in. A single exhalation should accompany this motion.

The rounded positioning of the arms, when performed with the correct expansion and contraction of the chest, can be compared with the opening and closing of a bear hug. *Caution:* The accurate execution of this movement requires a tucked in pelvis with the body weight concentrated on the heels and outer edges of the feet. Particular care should be taken to keep the knee over the toe of the weight-bearing leg.

Repeat the sequence of movement once more. Later you may progress to ten times in total. For an additional challenge, the lowest position can be held for five or six seconds with relaxed, continuous, deep breathing.

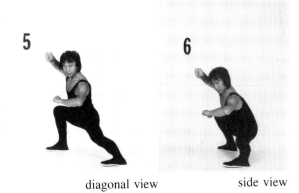

diagonal view   side view

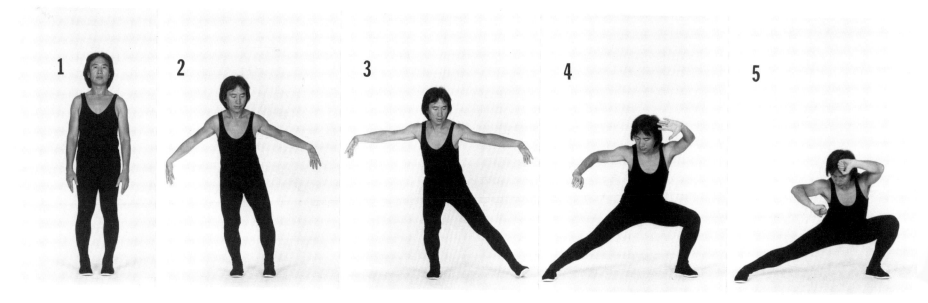

**Ninth Form:
Hitting the Tiger,
left side**

1) Stand in the neutral position with the feet parallel and narrower than the shoulder width. The breathing should be relaxed, continuous, and deep.

2) Begin to inhale a slow, deep breath. Tuck in the pelvis and shift the weight momentarily to the right leg. While turning the torso towards the left, step sideward with the left foot and bring the arms from the back to the front in a circular motion by using a contracting movement of the chest.

3, 4) With one fluid motion shift the weight again, this time to the left leg. Let the hips slowly sink down on the left leg and twist the upper torso towards the right. Continue to inhale the same breath.

5, 6) Loosely clench the fists as you bring the left arm up in an arc to the forehead and the right one in an arc to waist level. The rounded arms and the concave chest should form a smooth curve. Continue to sink down with the upper torso twisting toward the straightened right leg as you lean slightly forward. The right foot can slide outward as you sink down. Make sure the weight of the body is felt on the heel and outer edge of the left foot while taking care to align the left knee over the toes. It is important that this knee does not bend inward. The right foot should be resting flat on the ground, but carrying very little of the body's weight. The entire sinking down motion is rapid, about two to three seconds, and consists of a single inhalation.

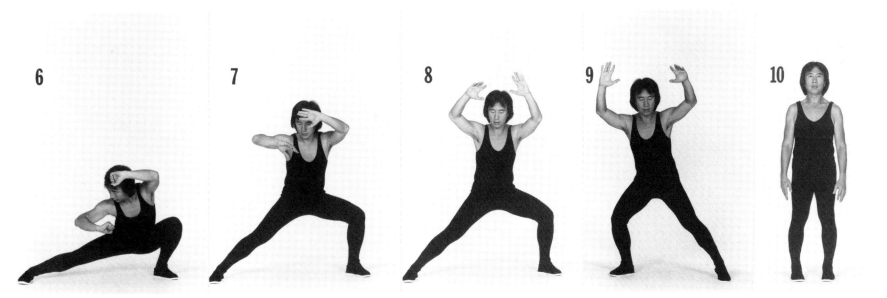

6   7   8   9   10

Make sure that the pelvis is still tucked in. Refer also to the side view and the diagonal view for the lowest position.

7, 8, 9, 10) In one fluid motion, return to the original position by pushing off the floor on the heel of the left foot, and reversing the previous arc of the arms. Again, make sure to keep the pelvis tucked in. A single exhalation should accompany this motion.

The rounded positioning of the arms, when performed with the correct expansion and contraction of the chest, can be compared with the opening and closing of a bear hug. *Caution:* The accurate execution of this movement requires a tucked in pelvis with the body weight concentrated on the heels and outer edges of the feet. Particular care should be taken to keep the knee over the toe of the weight-bearing leg.

Repeat the sequence of movement once more. Later you may progress to ten times in total. For an additional challenge, the lowest position can be held for five or six seconds with relaxed, continuous, deep breathing.

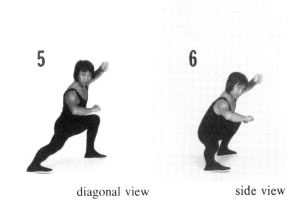

5   6

diagonal view   side view

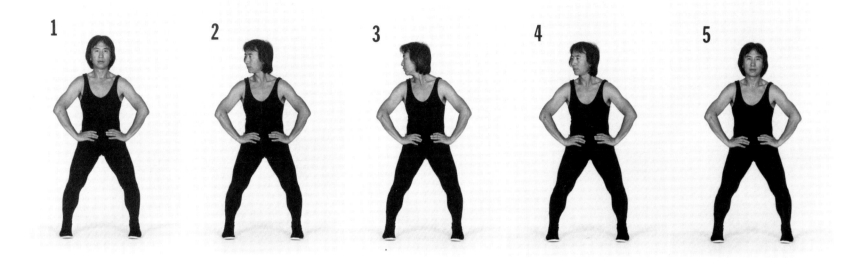

**Tenth Form:
Owl Turns Head**

1) Stand in the neutral position with the feet parallel and wider apart than the shoulder width. Let the body sink down by bending the knees and tucking in the pelvis. Turn the toes in slightly and spread the knees apart, focusing most of the body weight on the heels and outer edges of the feet. The weight should be distributed equally on each leg throughout this exercise. Place both hands on the hips, while the arms are kept rounded. Suspend the head. The breathing should be relaxed, continuous, and deep during this exercise.

2) Begin to slowly rotate the head to the right. Continue the rotation while keeping the torso and the hips facing forward. The head should be kept in the same horizontal plane throughout the rotation, which keeps the neck vertical.

3) At the furthest limit of rotation, hold for eight to ten seconds. Maintain a continuous stretching of the twisting neck at this point.

4, 5) Slowly rotate the head back to the center.

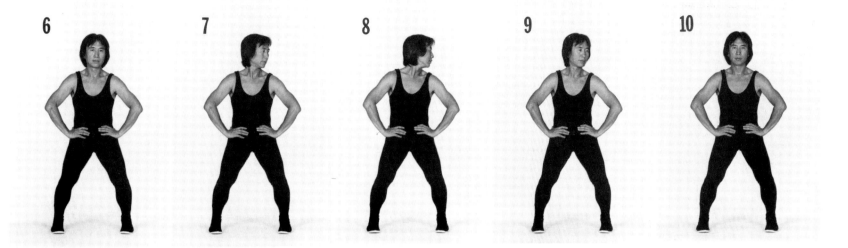

6, 7, 8, 9, 10) Continue the rotation to the left, again to its furthest extent. Hold for eight to ten seconds. Again, maintain the stretching of the neck. Return the head to a forward facing position. Repeat the entire sequence up to three more times.

Although this movement appears very simple, its subtlety is typical of the Nei Kung system. When analyzed on one level, for instance, it works on stretching an entire network of tendons throughout the body. Branches reach down the underside of the arms, through the palms, to the fingertips.

Likewise with the legs. All are connected through the back along the spine, which is being stretched and twisted the way you might wring out a wet washcloth.

Nei Kung Training Program

The following chart outlines my suggested Nei Kung training program. Although the progressive stages assume increasing stamina and ability, keep in mind that the correctness of the posture is the primary consideration.

This program is most effective when performed in its entirety and in the prescribed order. If your time is limited, start with Embracing Horse and proceed in order through the series as far as possible. It is better to spend more time on the first few movements than to try to rush through the entire set.

The advanced student should maintain the maximum durations listed while perfecting the details of the postures. For more intensive training, the frequency of sessions can be increased to once every other day, once a day, or even twice a day. There is virtually no limit to the benefit that can be reaped by the serious student.

Nei Kung Training Program	Start to 3 months	3 months to 6 months	6 months to 1 year	1 year to 2 years	2 years plus
I. Embracing Horse	3 min.	5 min.	8 min.	12 min.	15 min.
II. Riding the Wild Horse (middle, small, large)	2x	3x	4x	6x	6x
III. Playing P'i P'a (right, left)	.5 min.	1 min.	1.5 min.	2 min.	3 min.
IV. The Compass (right, left)	1x	2x	3x	4x	4x
V. Double Dragons Leap from Sea (right, left)	3x	4x	5x plus 10x fast	5x plus 10x fast	5x plus 10x fast
VI. Rhinoceros Gazes at the Moon	2x	2x	3x	4x	6x
VII. Riding Tiger (right, left)	1x	1x	2x	3x	3x
VIII. Phoenix Spreads Wings (forward, backward)	30x	30x	30x plus 10x fast	40x plus 10x fast	50x plus 20x fast
IX. Hitting the Tiger (right, left)	2x	2x	3x	4x	4x
X. Owl Turns Head	2x	2x	3x	4x	4x
Total time per session	approx. 20 min.	approx. 25 min.	approx. 40 min.	approx. 50 min.	approx. 60 min.
Number of sessions per week	2	2	2	3	3